I0420380

How to Make Yourself Beautiful in 10 Minutes

By

Robin Walton

Copyright © 2011, 2015 Robin Walton
All Rights Reserved
ISBN: 1517511089
ISBN-13: 978-1517511081

Table of Contents

Introduction

As the owner of a cosmetics company, it is my responsibility to not only provide my clients with the best and most diverse cosmetic line, but give my clients tips and advice that will enhance their natural beauty.

Many women think applying makeup is a long and tedious process. For some, the thought of applying makeup is considered a nightmare. Either way, women must choose to go all natural or save their makeup for a night on the town.

My book will put a stop to all doubt. When I say you can make yourself beautiful in ten minutes, I am not talking about lipstick and a pinch of blush. You will learn how to put on a day or night face in ten minutes with the help of personal and professional guidelines from me and various experts.

I know a ten-minute makeover can happen… I do it every day with products from my cosmetic line, Nestal Cosmetics®.

"How to Make Yourself Beautiful in 10 Minutes" will not only ease your doubts with tips on what colors and foundations work best with your complexion. Subsequently, expert advice on your skin and how to better care for your skin is also included.

Whether you are a business woman, stay at home mom, college student, or a woman with not enough time on your hands, my book will teach you how to take the time to make yourself beautiful.

After all at Nestal Cosmetics®: *"Our Number One Priority Is Your Beauty!"*®

- **Robin Walton, President and CEO of Nestal Cosmetics®**

Chapter I
How What You Eat Affects Your Skin

I am not a licensed physician, cosmetologist, or esthetician but I do know from personal experiences that what you eat can affect your inner health, physical health and skin.

One time, I went to my doctor for my regular check-up, blood work and all. When I returned for my test results, my doctor told me that my total cholesterol count was too high. She then suggested that I lose weight, stop eating fried foods, and exercise; that way she would not have to put me on medication. I followed my doctor's instructions and in a year, I lowered my cholesterol. My skin looked better, I looked better, and **NO MEDICATION WAS NEEDED!**

We must understand that eating the wrong foods can affect our bodies and skin. If you eat fried foods all of the time, it definitely causes problems such as heart disease, high blood pressure, and high cholesterol. Just as fried foods cause health problems, fried foods can also cause skin problems due to a lot of grease. The grease from fried foods are extracted through our skin and cause blemishes. Remember, this is coming out of the pores of your skin.

We must drink plenty of water; to cleanse the body of impurities and eliminate waste. A healthy diet is also suggested.

In addition, if you are a person who has problems with citric acid, then be careful with the citric fruits and juices. Try some vitamin supplements to get the nutrients that you need instead. I personally have an allergic reaction to oranges: one bite of a juicy orange causes my face to turn red and I breakout.

I love homemade lemonade but it does not like me. I will drink it maybe twice a week but I must make sure that I drink plenty of water afterwards in order to flush that good ole fashion lemonade out of my system.

The following is an excerpt from an article off of Essortment.com explaining, more so reinforcing my advice, on how to protect your skin. I hope it is as helpful to you as it has been to me.

How Diet Affects Your Skin

Healthy skin can be achieved through proper diet and by drinking plenty of water. Read on some tips to help improve your own skin.

(Information below provided by Essortment.com)

There are thousands of facial creams available on the market, each promising younger, smoother, more vibrant skin. And, while expensive creams and lotions can help soften the skin's surface, the basic foundation for healthy skin is good nutrition. Nothing can substitute for eating right in terms of overall health, and in particular, the tone and texture of one's skin.

One of the most important elements to achieving and maintaining healthy skin is drinking lots of water. Women are advised to drink at least eight glasses of water each day for a variety of reasons, and this practice is very beneficial for the skin. Water hydrates the cells of the skin, eliminating waste products, which in turn prevents constipation. This gives skin new softness and radiance. Additionally, keeping your skin hydrated will help to diminish lines and wrinkles, and eliminate pimples and blackheads.

Certain vitamins and minerals, specifically vitamins A, C, and E are beneficial to skin as well. Iron can also contribute to healthy skin tone. People with vitamin deficiencies tend to have skin that is dry and does not heal properly. Many people tend to have particularly dry skin in the winter when harsh, cold air combines with a lack of sunshine, which provides vitamin C. Very dry skin, especially on the hands and feet, can crack and even bleed.

B1 vitamins are particularly helpful. B1 keeps circulation normal, which in turn contributes to healthy skin. B2 can actually eliminate aging spots on the skin, while B6 helps prevent eczema. Brewer's yeast is a natural source of B vitamins. Ingest two tablespoons of dried brewer's yeast each day for two weeks, and you will see a noticeable difference in skin tone.

Fiber is also important in maintaining healthy skin. As with water, eating fiber prevents constipation, which in turn can be detrimental to skin health. To get more fiber, consider eating more apples and include whole grains in your diet. Simply changing from white rice to brown rice will increase fiber intake. Add beans to the rice and you have a high fiber, low fat main course. Other good sources of fiber are cauliflower and broccoli. Look for snacks that are high in fiber such as nuts, dates, figs, raisins, and seeds.

Eating fish can also be very beneficial to your complexion. The oils in fish will actually help to feed moisture to your skin. It is suggested that at least one meal per day include some type of fish, either fresh or canned. Even canned tuna qualifies in this department!

Flaxseeds are another readily available food source that can help maintain healthy skin. Ground up, flaxseeds contain what is known as omega-three fatty acids, which are highly beneficial to skin health. Some special diets suggest sprinkling flaxseed over your cereal or adding to yogurt.

Don't forget dairy products, especially milk, and make sure to include vegetable oils in your diet along with yogurts. Always avoid junk food as much as possible. Snacks such as candy, chips, crackers, cookies, and cakes are high in fat and calories, and also can be loaded with salt which has a counter-effect to drinking water.

Combining good nutrition with a sensible exercise program and plenty of rest can make an enormous difference in overall skin health. Fancy creams can make you feel better, but the essentials of good skin care come down to some very elemental basics that are so simple, anyone can do them. Just remember, drink lots of water! You won't be sorry!

Chapter II
Washing Your Face

Learning to wash your face properly is very important, but it is especially essential to those who wear makeup. You want to make sure you clean your face properly. There are face cleansers and mild soaps. I personally use soap made from oatmeal; it cleans well, it's mild and does not dry out my skin, and I use this soap over my entire body.

Some soaps will leave an oily build up on your skin, which can cause your skin to be dry and that causes break outs.

After finding a good cleanser and toner, to remove any excess makeup and dirt from your face, you must also moisturize your face, whether it is normal, oily, or dry. You can find these items and more on my website, **www.nestalcosmetics.com**

There are different skin types:

Normal: Normal skin is smooth and even in texture, healthy in color.

Combination: Combination skin is part normal and oily together. You may find after a while that oil comes through the T-Zone, the area around the nose, forehead and around the eyes.

Oily: Oily Skin is just what it says. Oil comes from the pores of your skin which causes blackheads and blemishes on your face.

Sensitive: Sensitive skin tends to be thin and delicate. It easily breaks out and forms a rash.

Dry: Dry skin feels tight after washing. It may flake and has red patches on it.

Now here are some tips on the proper technique for washing your face from Dr. Anne Dacko, a certified dermatologist in New York City. She wrote these tips for About.com.

How to Wash Your Face Properly

With Dr. Anne Dacko for About.com

If you want blackhead free skin, you need to properly wash your face. Learn the best technique for washing your face and maintaining your youthful grow.

Hello, my name is Dr. Anne Dacko. I'm a certified dermatologist here in New York City and I'm here for About.com.

Why Wash Your Face?

Today we're going to talk about the importance and the proper technique for washing your face. Using a proper technique to wash your face is very important so that you maintain a youthful appearance of your skin and also so that you can prevent blackheads and wrinkling of the skin.

I'm going to tell you the proper technique for washing your face.

Wet Your Face

First, you put a headband on to pull the hair out of your face. And then you gently take water, warm water, and splash it on your face.

Apply Cleanser

Then take a gently facial cleanser. Pour out a small amount on your hands. Rub it together and in gentle circular motion rub it on your face. Don't forget to go close to your hairline, your forehead, and gently over your eyelids and mouth. And then take cool or warm water and gently splash it on your face to rinse. Then with a towel, gently pat your face dry.

Apply Moisturizer

And then you apply a facial moisturizer, preferably something with an SPF 15 or 30 in order to protect your skin and seal in any moisture and prevent sun damage.

If you follow this technique, you will have healthier and younger looking skin.

Chapter III
Matching Your Skin Tone

When buying clothes we all try to buy colors that look good on us. There is also colors we should stay away from. Dark green is a color that does absolutely nothing for me. So when it comes to choosing foundation and powders, we must find the correct shade for our skin tone.

I've watched people, and I also have been guilty of this in the past, try to match powder and foundation by applying it to the back of their hands or the inside of their wrists. Well that does not work; the back of your hands and the inside of your wrists are not the same color as your face. When matching color for your fact you want to test the powder or foundation on your lower jaw line.   if the color blends naturally, then you are in business. In addition, let's be careful with choosing foundation and powders in a poorly lit room.

For ladies who love to wear off the shoulder and low cut tops, but have surgical scars, blemishes, or have vitiligo, I have just the cover up that you need. It's called Paramedical Kamaflage. This camouflage makeup comes in various shades that match every skin tone. After applying this cream, use an Oil Free Pressed Powder or Two-way Foundation to set the cream.

Magnificent!

Here at Nestal Cosmetics®, we want to enhance your beauty by making sure you look natural and beautiful. Our Number One Priority Is Your Beauty! ®

When picking eye shadows, you want to stay with natural colors until you learn and experiment with other colors. Try lipsticks and lip glosses that best suits you. When using lip liners or lip pencils, be sure to get the ones that match your lipstick or lip gloss color. These items are used to prevent your lipstick or lip gloss from bleeding.

When it comes to picking blush, if you are not sure about the color, go with something natural. You will be surprised on how this will accent your cheeks.

Eyebrow pencils and eyeliners should match your hair color; black and brown would be a good choice. Black mascara looks great on all lashes. I have very thin eyebrows and as I get older, they get even thinner. Over the years I have had to draw my brows with a pencil and I have done well with lots of practice. However, since eyebrow pencils have wax and this causes eyebrows to shine. I learned a little trick from Mr. Sam Fine, the world famous makeup artist. Apply a small amount of eye shadow that is lighter than the eye pencil prevents shining, thus creating the natural look. Thank you, Mr. Fine.

Ladies, let's not forget to get our eyebrows professionally arched, waxed, threaded, or tweezed. Doing so will change your whole appearance and afterwards you'll look at yourself and say, "Wow!"

Now that we have covered the basics, we will start our final chapter on "How to Make Yourself Beautiful in 10 Minutes."

Chapter IV
Let's Get Started

Remember to moisturize your face whether it is washing your face before going to bed at night or after showering in the morning. I'm sure that you have also picked out what you will be wearing the night before. Therefore, your makeup should be in a place where it is easy to get.

When applying your powder or foundation with your cosmetic wedge, use your Powder Brush or your Kabuki Brush to blend your makeup.

Afterwards, it is now time to apply your blush:

1. Look into the mirror and smile. You are smiling because all of us don't have perfect cheekbones. Doing this will help you apply your blush in the correct area of your face.
2. Start at the hairline at the above opening of your ears with your wedge sponge
3. Apply the blush across your cheek, stopping before you get to your nose.
4. Take your Kabuki Brush or Blush Brush and blend your blush. Do not make circles on your cheeks.

Now it is time to apply your eye liner or eye pencil:

1. Start with the inside corner of your eye to the outside corner. If you want to do the upper eye lid, line it in the same way.
2. Anytime you are lining your lower eye lid, use your middle finger to pull it down; this finger puts less pressure on the skin below the eye, helping to prevent hard wrinkling under the eye.
3. Add a little mascara using upward strokes

If you have those eyebrows in order as I suggested, then you won't have too much to do with them, just add a little eye pencil.

Lastly, you are ready to take care of your lips:

1. Be sure to follow your natural lip line when lining your lips
2. Apply your lipstick or lip gloss.

Your face is now done in **10 MINUTES!**

Whether you are going out for the evening or if it is one of your days off from work, you can experiment a little more on making yourself look beautiful. Enjoy ladies and email me at **robin@nestalcosmetics.com** or at **info@nestalcosmetics.com** to let me know how you did. If you wish to make purchases visit my website at **www.nestalcosmetics.com** and click on the online store. Visa, MasterCard or Discover are accepted.

I look forward to hearing from you.

Easy Makeup Tools

Powder Brush

Blush Brush

Sponges (Cosmetic Wedges, latex-free to be safe)

Kabuki Brush (my favorite)

Shadow Brush

Sharpener (for eyebrow pencils & lip pencils)

You may add these later:

Angle Brush

Lip Brush

Contour Brush

Blender

Purchase a good set of brushes and they will last a long time. Brushes made from sable and pony hair are my favorites. They can be washed with regular hand soap just be sure to rinse them well and then let them air dry.

Please don't share your makeup tools with others.

Customer Testimonials

Dear Robin,

Thank you so very much for the makeover. I went through a major life change that was only enhanced by the cosmetics that I purchased. I went to my 25 year class reunion and I felt like the Belle of the Ball. I had so much more confidence that I have experienced in years. The product is very light and wears well. I love the looks of approval and the verbal compliments that I always get when wearing my new face! I wish you every success in the future with Nestal Cosmetics®!!!!!!!!!!!!!!!!!!!!!!!!!

D. Oliver; Arlington, TX

Dear Robin,

The book was great and full of useful information. I like the tip on how to properly wash your face. I've also discovered that I actually have combination skin instead of normal like I always thought. My skin is part normal and oily, especially in the T-Zone areas of my face. The nutritional tips were great too, like drinking more water. This book is a great reference book, not to read just once. Thanks Sister Robin for this book.

M. English; Merrillville, IN

Hi, Mrs. Walton!

First let me say I love love love the Sensitive Skin Solutions products you recommended. My skin looks more alive since I've been using the Sensitive face wash, toner, and Vitamin E Crème. After reading your book "How to Make Yourself Beautiful in 10 Minutes", I realize I was doing so many things wrong. From the way I wash my face, the things I eat and drink, and how I apply makeup. Your book informed me that keeping up beauty is simple, fun, and easy. Doing a few steps daily makes all the difference in how our skin looks and feels. And we all want to look and feel great. Thank you for sharing your knowledge.

Be blessed mighty woman of God!

Tiffany; Houston, TX

If you are looking for make-up that enhances the natural beauty of your skin, then you have found it in Nestal Cosmetics®. I absolutely love Nestal Cosmetics® oil free press powder/two-way foundation because it feels light and looks so natural on my skin. And, because I prefer to look "naturally enhanced" as opposed to "made-up", I made the switch after one make-over and have not looked back. Friends and family have noted the difference with compliments that support the goal of my make-up application such as, "You look so beautiful and so natural", and want to know my secret. So, I am sharing my secret with you. Moreover, the education provided by founder of Nestal Cosmetics®, Robin Walton, on makeup application during my make-over has been invaluable to me. I am excited that I no longer have to ask someone else to put eye shadow on for me--I can now do it myself when I want to wear it. And thanks to Nestal Cosmetics® color phase eye shadow, I no longer concern over the complimentary colors to create subtle or dramatic eyes. So, thanks Robin for the education and the color phase eye shadow. So go for it and get your make-over with Nestal Cosmetics® as I am convinced that you too will become a user.

Connie Martin; Gary, IN

I am a big fan of Nestal's "Berry Sexy" lipstick. Needless to say, when I wear it I do look very sexy, and I am often complimented on the shade. I also love the powdered eye shadows they blend very well for a natural look that is very complementing to the eyes. I love Nestal Cosmetics®, I recommend them to my friends on a regular basis and I am a customer for life.

Thank you Robin for Nestal Cosmetics®!

Cheryl D. Wiggins; Griffith, IN

I have been a long time customer of Nestal Cosmetics® and I love the products because I DO NOT get an allergic reaction to any of the makeup items I have purchased from the company. And because my skin has switched from oily to combination skin over the years, Nestal Cosmetics® foundation works perfectly because it does not leave my face oily or shiny once I apply it. I also love lipstick and one of my favorite lipsticks is Hypnotic because it complements my lips. I would encourage all women to give Nestal Cosmetics a try; it is well worth the reasonable price!

L. DeNeal; Gary, IN

About the Author

Robin Walton is President and CEO of Nestal Cosmetics®. She is a wife and mother of 2 adult sons, a native Gary, IN. Robin is also a Christian Baptist who received a vision from God in 2006 to start her own business. Robin enjoys helping other people who are in need of uplifting. She has partnered with non-profit organizations in the business of uplifting women who have been in risky and challenging situations.

In addition, Robin answered her calling and as of January 8, 2014 is an Ordained Christian Minister; and presiding over her son's wedding later that year on May 25, 2014.

Her company motto is Our Number One Priority Is Your Beauty!®. When she speaks of this she is not only speaking of your outer beauty but she speaks on your inner beauty as well. She was inspired to write "How to Make Yourself Beautiful in 10 Minutes" after listening to so many women say that they never have time to put on makeup or that they do not know how to apply it.

"I do hope you enjoy my book and it gives you exactly what you need to Make Yourself Beautiful in 10 Minutes

-   Robin Walton, President & CEO, Nestal Cosmetics®

Visit my website at **www.nestalcosmetics.com** for all your cosmetic needs

Nestal Cosmetics®
4021 E. 13th Ave
Gary, IN 46403
866-713-6114

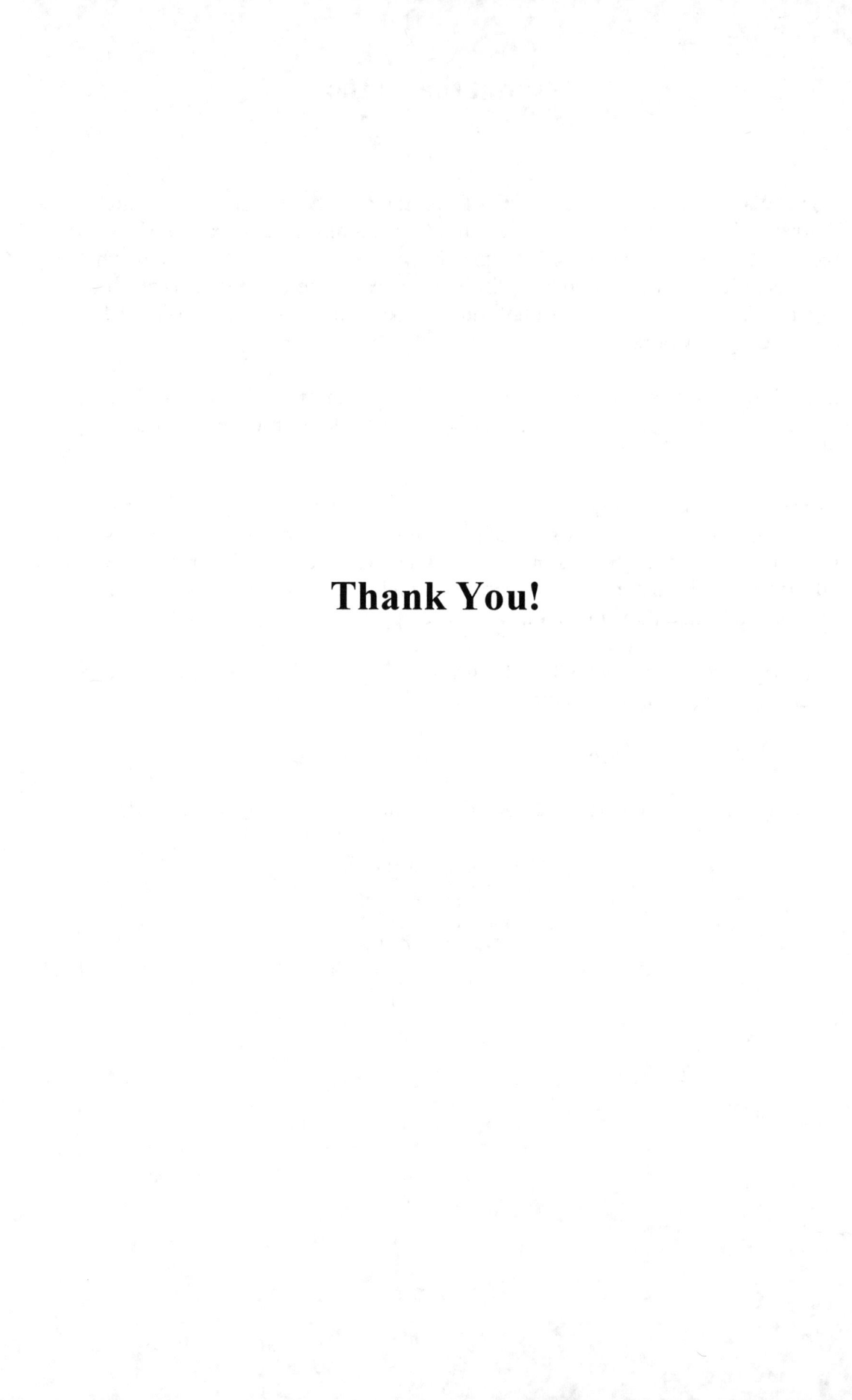

Thank You!

www.ingramcontent.com/pod-product-compliance
Lightning Source LLC
Chambersburg PA
CBHW081143280526
45787CB00007B/3201